Hèla Ben Jmaà
Fatma Mhiri
Salma Charfeddine

Beating heart coronary bypass surgery

Hèla Ben Jmaà
Fatma Mhiri
Salma Charfeddine

Beating heart coronary bypass surgery

Beating heart myocardial revascularization

ScienciaScripts

Imprint

Any brand names and product names mentioned in this book are subject to trademark, brand or patent protection and are trademarks or registered trademarks of their respective holders. The use of brand names, product names, common names, trade names, product descriptions etc. even without a particular marking in this work is in no way to be construed to mean that such names may be regarded as unrestricted in respect of trademark and brand protection legislation and could thus be used by anyone.

Cover image: www.ingimage.com

This book is a translation from the original published under ISBN 978-620-6-72192-5.

Publisher:
Sciencia Scripts
is a trademark of
Dodo Books Indian Ocean Ltd. and OmniScriptum S.R.L publishing group

120 High Road, East Finchley, London, N2 9ED, United Kingdom
Str. Armeneasca 28/1, office 1, Chisinau MD-2012, Republic of Moldova, Europe
Printed at: see last page
ISBN: 978-620-8-08206-2

BEATING HEART CORONARY BYPASS SURGERY

I- INTRODUCTION

Coronary artery disease is the leading cause of death worldwide, and myocardial revascularisation is the best treatment for atheromatous lesions of the coronary arteries.

Systolic heart failure (HF), currently defined as a fall in left ventricular ejection fraction (LVEF) below 40%, can be a complication of coronary artery disease. It currently represents a major public health problem due to its frequency and severity in terms of mortality and morbidity (1).

The prevalence of CI is 1 to 2% of the general population (2). This prevalence is increasing as life expectancy rises and the population ages.

In developing countries such as Tunisia, CI has a major economic impact as it affects a younger, more active population.
(3). Health expenditure attributed to heart failure remains high because of its direct cost (high number of hospitalisations, cost of pharmacological and interventional treatment) and indirect cost (social and professional handicap) (4).

Patients with impaired systolic left ventricular ejection fraction (LVEF) of ischaemic origin, in the absence of surgical or interventional myocardial revascularisation, have a poor prognosis with a two-year survival of around 31% when they progress to congestive heart failure (2).

Coronary artery bypass grafting (CABG) is the gold standard of treatment compared with medical therapy in patients with left ventricular (LV) systolic dysfunction with left common trunk (LCT) or tritruncal involvement (1, 5-8).

The aims of myocardial revascularisation in coronary patients with left ventricular dysfunction are to improve ventricular function, prevent congestive heart failure and improve the quality of life and life expectancy of these patients.

Compared with patients with preserved LVEF, left ventricular dysfunction increases the risk of surgery (9). This makes the choice of operative strategy all the more important in reducing intra- and post-operative morbidity and mortality. Extracorporeal circulation (ECG) has been one of the most significant advances in medicine and its implementation has made modern cardiac surgery safe and effective. Beating heart coronary surgery is one of the techniques used in cases of left ventricular dysfunction. Its introduction was largely based on avoiding the complications associated with bypass surgery.

However, despite advances in interventional cardiology and surgical techniques, in-hospital mortality in patients with impaired left ventricular function remains high compared with patients with preserved LV function (6-8).

The debate therefore remains open as to the best method of surgical or endovascular myocardial revascularisation, and the place of beating heart surgery in these fragile patients (6).

Theoretical advantages of CB surgery include the possibility of reducing blood transfusions, postoperative hospital length of stay, postoperative neurocognitive decline and systemic anticoagulation (10). Observational studies have also suggested that CB surgery significantly reduces mortality and morbidity compared with CABG.

II- INCIDENCE OF CORONARY ARTERY DISEASE WITH IMPAIRED LVEF

Heart failure may be the result of myocardial or valvular pathology, pericardial, endocardial or rhythmic. Several classifications of heart failure have been proposed. We have retained the classification of heart failure based on LVEF, which distinguishes between heart failure with reduced ejection fraction (rEF) and heart failure with preserved ejection fraction (pEF).

CHF with rEF (also known as systolic CHF) is defined as the presence of a left ventricular ejection fraction < 40%. Heart attack with pEF (also known as diastolic heart attack) is defined as the presence of an ejection fraction $\geq$ 50%, associated with a structural anomaly (1).

Table I: Distribution of the average age of patients having undergone bypass surgery coronary artery disease with left ventricular dysfunction, depending on the series.

Study	Years	Age groups	Average age
Elefteriades et al (11)	1986-1992	42 to 83 years	66.8 years old
Kron et al (12)	1983-1988	43 to 80 years	63.3 years old
Hillis et al (13)	1995-1999	61 to 79 years old	69 years old
Wu et al (14)	1991-2002	38 to 86 years	67.9 years old
Wang et al (15)	2013-2017	-	61 years old

Table II: Sex distribution of patients having undergone coronary bypass with left ventricular dysfunction according to series.

Study	Years	Male sex (%)
Elefteriades et al (11)	1986-1992	83,13
Kron et al (12)	1983-1988	79,48
Hillis et al (13)	1995-1999	76
Wu et al (14)	1991-2002	92,1
Wang et al (15)	2013-2017	70,5

A history of coronary heart disease has also been found in several studies (16, 17). In a study by Nagendran et al in 2013 (16), 90% of patients had a history of acute coronary events of which 4% had a history of TCA and 1% had a history of CABG. Nagendran et al (16) noted the presence of a history of peripheral vascular disease in 14.2% of the population studied, and a history of stroke in 10.1%.

III-CLINICAL STUDY

1- Circumstances of discovery :

Coronary insufficiency can manifest itself in a number of clinical pictures, ranging from silent ischaemia to acute coronary syndrome with or without electrical changes, or even heart failure (18).

In a study published by Nagendran et al (17) including 2837 patients, the clinical presentation was dominated by ACS (61%), followed by stable angina (30%). However, the study by Algarni et al (19) showed that the dominant clinical presentation in 5364 patients was stable angina (37.2%), followed by ST- ACS (31.3%), and ST+ ACS (23.3%).

Preoperative congestive heart failure was described in 66.6% of patients in the series by Kron et al (12), and in 52% of patients in the series by Elefteriades et al (11).

In a recent study involving 112 patients, Wang et al (15) reported dyspnoea in 77% of patients. In another study by Wu et al (14) including 3308 patients, dyspnoea was found in 57.8% of cases.

2- Physical and para-clinical examination :

The physical examination may also reveal signs of left heart failure or pulmonary oedema, or abnormalities associated with peripheral vascular damage associated with coronary artery disease.

The ECG is usually abnormal, revealing signs of ischaemia and/or sequelae of myocardial infarction. On the other hand, a normal ECG can be seen in 20% of cases, and cannot exclude coronary pathology, which is in favour of the poor sensitivity of this test. The study of hibernating myocardium using dobutamine ultrasound and myocardial scintigraphy is of great importance in assessing the reversibility of left ventricular dysfunction after restoration of coronary perfusion. These investigations systematically look for myocardial viability, and make it possible to select patients who are candidates for myocardial revascularisation in the event of severe ventricular dysfunction.

Pre-operative TTE, in addition to studying pre-operative LVEF, makes it possible to assess segmental kinetics and PAPS, and to look for any associated valve damage.

Coronary angiography is the gold standard for diagnosing coronary lesions. It is used to assess the location and degree of stenoses, the condition of the downstream bed, to establish coronary status and the Syntax score, and to determine the indication for revascularisation.

All the authors noted in their studies a majority of tritroncular lesions associated or not with damage to the TCG.

Studies in the literature have shown that mortality rates were similar in the two groups of patients who underwent percutaneous revascularisation or CABG, and who had coronary anatomy of low to intermediate complexity measured by the Syntax score ($\leq$32).

The various coronary lesions analysed were :

- Stage of stenosis: This has been defined with reference to the classification of the American College of Cardiology and the American Heart Association (ACC/AHA).

Patients are classified as mono-, bi- or tri-truncular depending on whether the main axes (anterior interventricular (AIV), circumflex (Cx) or right coronary artery (RCA)) or their collaterals (diagonal (Dg), marginal (Mg), posterior interventricular (PVI) or left retroventricular (LVR) respectively) are involved.

- Severity of stenosis :

•A stenosis is considered significant if it is $\geq$ 50% at the level of the left coronary trunk (LCT), or at the level of the ostial IVA, and $\geq$ 70% at the level of other arteries of diameter ≥ 1.5 millimetres (mm).

• A chronic coronary occlusion corresponds to a complete interruption of anterograde blood flow in a coronary artery, and on coronary angiography corresponds to a TIMI 0 flow (Thrombolysis In Myocardial Infarction). This obstruction must have been present for at least three months.

• Analysis of coronary flow: A classification developed by the TIMI study team distinguished 4 types of flow (14) (Appendix 3).

- The SYNTAX Score I anatomical risk score is calculated in the event of TCG involvement or associated tritruncal involvement.

IV-INDICATIONS FOR BEATING HEART BYPASS SURGERY: 1-MONOTRUNCAL LESIONS

According to the 2018 revascularisation recommendations (20), in the case of ostio-proximal IVA involvement the CABG is recommended in class IA. PCB could be a good alternative for the treatment of this type of lesion.

 BLAZEK et al (21), in a study spanning 7 years, demonstrated that stenting or MIDCAB surgery for isolated proximal LAI lesions was associated with similar long-term results in terms of the endpoints (death from cardiac causes and myocardial infarction).

2- Impaired LV function :

According to European guidelines for myocardial revascularisation, CABG is an alternative of choice in multi-truncular patients with LV dysfunction $\leq 35\%$ (20). PCB is a good therapeutic option in these patients.

A meta-analysis concluded that PCB may be associated with lower early mortality in patients with impaired left ventricular function.

3- Elderly patients with co-morbidities :

Theoretical considerations and the results of retrospective studies have suggested that postoperative morbidity may be reduced when CABG is performed without CEC. Advances in surgical techniques, the use of intra-coronary shunts and improvements in epicardial stabilisation devices have made it easier for surgeons to perform multi-patient CABG (22).

PCB has become increasingly popular over the last decade among octogenarians. The renewed interest in beating heart surgery is associated with the belief that the deleterious effects of the pump can be avoided, leading to better outcomes and potentially reduced costs and use of resources (23).

4- PCBs and co-morbidities :

The PCB makes it possible to avoid aortic manipulation, which can be a potential source of atheromatous embolisms that can lead to significant neurological complications (24, 25).

5- Revascularisation surgery of the left common trunk :

CABG is the revascularisation method of choice for patients with TCG stenosis, especially if associated with a SYNTAX I score $\geq$ 23 (20). Revascularisation surgery without CEC, in cases of TCG stenosis, is a safe alternative to surgery under CEC (26).

However, the beating heart surgical treatment of tight lesions of the TCG was at one time considered to be a relative contraindication, in relation to the haemodynamic disturbances that occur when the heart is dislocated during this surgical procedure. At present, haemodynamic disturbances have been reduced by technological advances and improved anaesthetic techniques and procedures, making this method of revascularisation safer.

6- Redux surgery:

Re-operation for bypass surgery in a patient who has already undergone revascularisation and/or valve replacement surgery can be extremely difficult. The adhesions that have formed can make it difficult to control the old bypasses (when they are still permeable) and to dissect the posterior wall of the heart (27).

V- MEDICAL TREATMENT

In the series by Elefteriades et al involving coronary bypass surgery in patients with LVEF < 30%, an intra-aortic counterpulsation balloon was placed pre-operatively in 19% of patients for low cardiac output, and in 43% of patients prophylactically to maintain a stable haemodynamic state during surgery and facilitate weaning from the CEC (11). Since its publication in 2011, the Euroscore II has been the most widely used risk score in Europe for patients undergoing cardiac surgery. In the literature, the STS score underestimates predicted mortality when compared with the Euroscore II. It is around 1.2 with extremes between 0.7 and 2.3.

VI-ANAESTHESIA PROTOCOL

Pre-anaesthetic management involves fasting for at least 6 hours and the administration of an oral anxiolytic premedication, hydroxyzine (ATARAX) at a dose of 1mg/kg the day before the operation and two hours before arrival in the operating theatre.The β-blockers, nitrates and calcium channel blockers are continued until the morning of the operation, while the other cardiovascular treatments are stopped the day before. Other treatments are continued or stopped in accordance with the usual recommendations. In the operating theatre, patients are positioned supine on a mattress. heated to prevent hypothermia. Once the intra-operative monitoring equipment has been installed, a catheter is inserted into the radial artery for continuous blood pressure monitoring and blood sampling. After pre-oxygenation, anaesthesia is induced using intravenous agents. It uses a combination of a hypnotic (ethomidate) 0.2 mg/kg, a morphine analgesic (Remifentanyl) (Ultiva*) 1.5 mg/kg over one minute) and a curarising agent (Cisatracurium) (Nimbex) 0.2 mg/kg). After orotracheal intubation, patients are ventilated in controlled mode with a 50% oxygen/air mixture and a tidal volume of 8 to 10 ml/kg to maintain a $PaCO_2$ between 35 and 40 mm Hg. Maintenance of anaesthesia is ensured by a combination of propofol 6 mg/kg/hour Remifentanyl 0.2 to 0.4 µg/kg/min and Cisatracurium 0.1 mg/kg/h. Intraoperative monitoring includes a 5-lead ECG, pulsatile oxygen saturation, invasive blood pressure, capnogram, central venous pressure, biological monitoring with blood gas, renal function, blood ionogram, blood count and diuresis.Antibiotic prophylaxis consists of intravenous injections of 1.5 g of Zinnat after induction and 750 mg every 4 hours throughout the operation, then every 8 hours for the first 24 hours. In cases of allergy or high risk of colonisation by multi-resistant Staphylococcus aureus, Vancomycin 15 mg/kg is administered IV over one hour at induction. A dose of heparin is injected by the anaesthetist into the central catheter, to achieve an activated clotting time of more than 400 seconds.

VII- SURGICAL TECHNIQUES

CABG surgery is the gold standard for myocardial revascularisation in coronary patients with left ventricular dysfunction (5). In the majority of cases, patients with TCG stenosis underwent surgery. rapidly, except in cases of extreme emergency. Several authors have studied the evolution of these patients in the days leading up to the operation in order to determine the factors with a poor prognosis and to identify the indications for urgent surgery. They concluded that surgery should be performed within the first 10 days following catheterisation in patients with severe symptoms or recent myocardial infarction.

1- Approach :

The approach may be a vertical median sternotomy, or a left anterior mini-thoracotomy (Minimally invasive direct access coronary artery bypass "MID CAB").

1-1- Median sternotomy :

The median sternotomy allows good visualisation of the coronary arteries and internal mammary arteries, and easy dislocation of the heart so that coronary anastomoses can be performed correctly (28).

1-2- Left anterior mini-thoracotomy :

The "MID CAB" technique involves bypassing a coronary artery located directly under the incision, usually via a left anterior mini-thoracotomy. The left internal mammary artery is isolated from the chest wall under direct vision, and more recently video-assisted, and is then sutured to the VIA while the heart is beating (29). This technique was initially developed in countries where the number of bypass operations was limited for economic reasons (30).

Left anterior mini-thoracotomy at the level of the fifth intercostal space allows access to the anterior interventricular, diagonal and proximal right coronary arteries (31, 32).

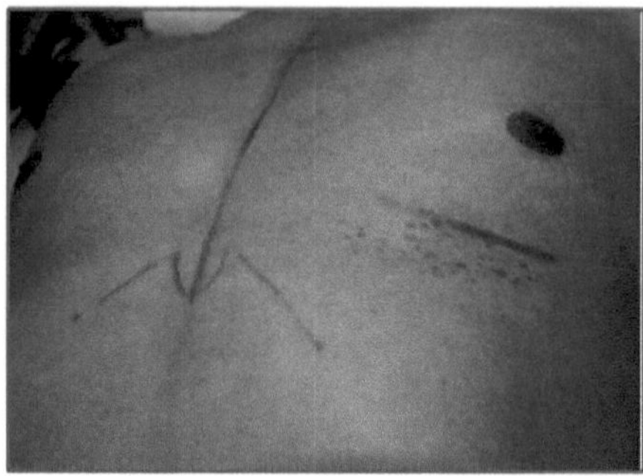

Figure 1: Anatomical landmarks for left anterior mini-thoracotomy (32).

1- 3- Right anterior mini-thoracotomy :

Occasionally, the right internal mammary artery has been used to revascularise the DC via a right anterior mini-thoracotomy (33).

2- Choice of graft :

The left internal mammary artery graft, used since the 1960s, is now considered to be the graft of choice for coronary artery bypass grafting, especially for revascularisation of the VIA (34). The right internal mammary artery, although theoretically having the same properties as the AMIG, is less frequently used. It can be used as a pedicle or as a free graft. The free graft is mainly used to reach a segment of the coronary artery that is distal enough for a pedicled graft. The saphenous graft, reimplanted on the ascending aorta, can be used to revascularise the diagonal, marginal and right coronary arteries.

3- Beating heart surgery technique :

3- 1- MIDCAB technique :

The left internal mammary artery (LIMMA), isolated from the chest wall under direct vision, and more recently video-assisted, is then sutured with a beating heart to the VIA (32, 35).

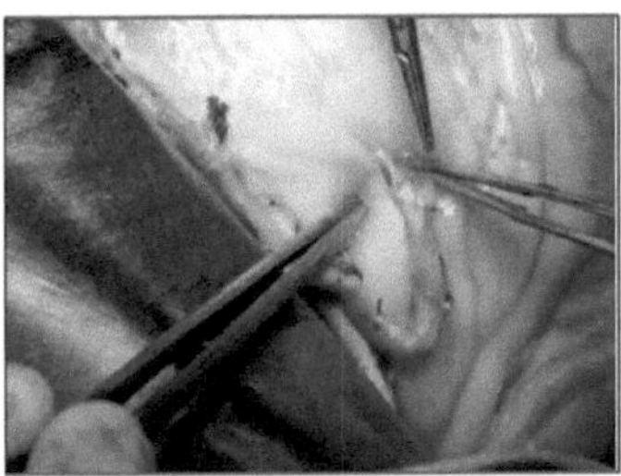

Figure 2: End-to-side anastomosis between the AMIG and the IVA.

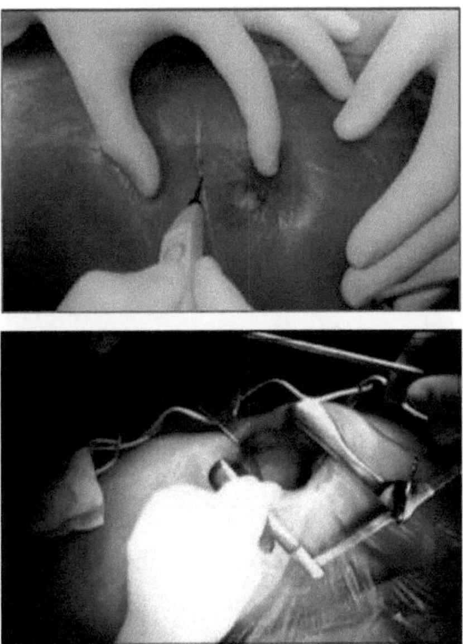

Figures 3 and 4: MIDCAB AMIG IVA bypass surgery.

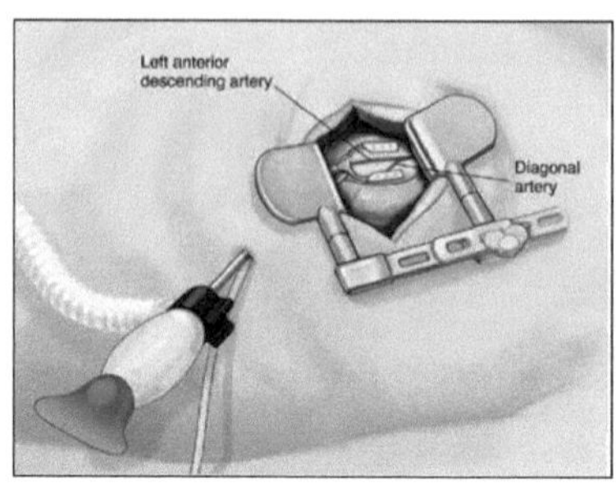

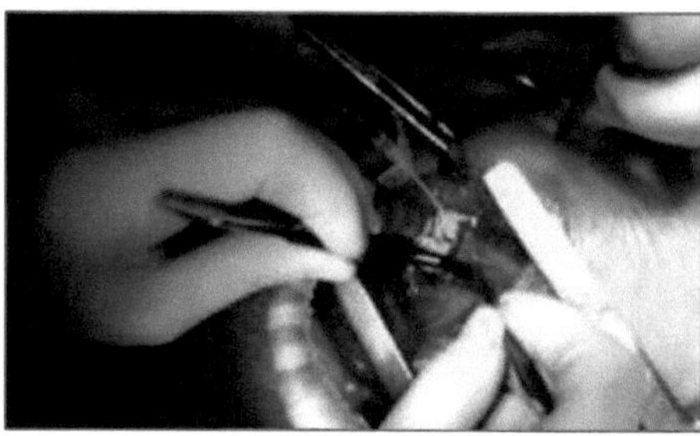

Figures 5 and 6: Beating heart IVA anastomosis using the MIDCAB technique (32).

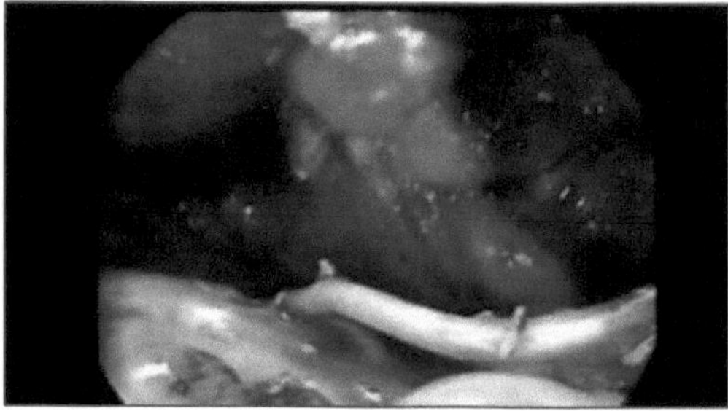

Figure 7: AMIG anastomosis on the left IVA performed by MIDCAB.

In the study carried out by Arslan et al (36), the authors found that, compared with patients operated on with PCB by sternotomy, patients operated on with MIDCAB had a significantly shorter duration of mechanical ventilation, a shorter duration of stay in the intensive care unit and in hospital, and required fewer blood transfusions. Florisson et al (37) concluded that MIDCAB was associated with higher morbidity and a higher reoperation rate than PCB via sternotomy, but the two techniques were equivalent in terms of operative and medium-term mortality. However, this technique can only be proposed for patients with only one or two blood vessels. and requires a learning curve on the part of the cardiac surgeon before perform coronary anastomoses under more difficult conditions than during conventional coronary surgery by sternotomy and with CEC (38).

3- 2- Technique of surgery à heart beating heart by median sternotomy :

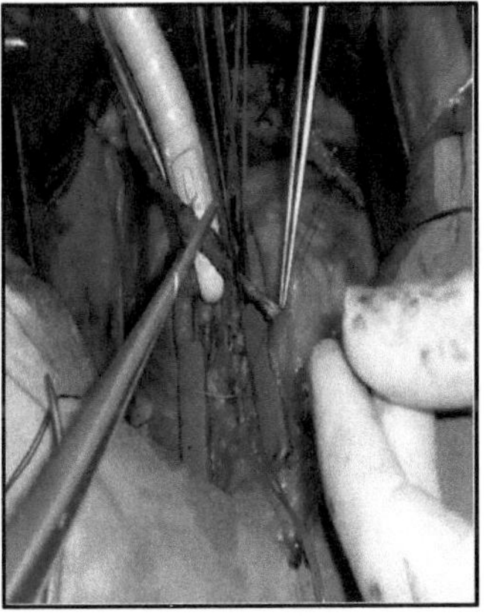

Figure 8: Anastomosis between the IVA and the AMIG during bypass with CB.

VIII- ADVANTAGES AND LIMITATIONS OF BEATING HEART SURGERY:

1- Advantages

Beating heart aorto-coronary bypass surgery has been performed for over 30 years (38). The consequences o f intra-operative myocardial ischaemia and the specific side-effects of bypass surgery have led to the development of beating heart bypass techniques in patients with left ventricular dysfunction. Avoiding the use of the cardiopulmonary bypass circuit would considerably reduce the diffuse systemic inflammatory response during and after surgery. cardiac surgery. This reduces platelet activation and changes in the coagulation and fibrinolytic systems (39).

Recourse to cardioplegic arrest and associated ischaemia-reperfusion lesions is also avoided (40). Technological advances and improved anaesthetic techniques and procedures have also reduced haemodynamic disturbances during bypass surgery, making this method of revascularisation safer.Pres ervation of pulsatile flow, preservation of normal movements of the interventricular septum, even improvement in septal contractility as a result of revascularisation, and better post-operative blood flow in breast grafts due to the absence of post-CEC myocardial oedema are also advantages of beating heart surgery (41, 42).

Beating heart coronary anastomoses must be performed using cardiac stabilisation systems to revascularise as many coronary territories as possible. These stabilisers may be compression-based or suction-based using the Octopus system.

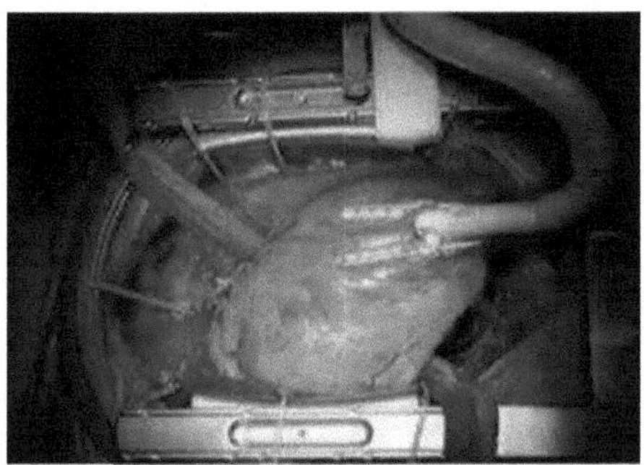

Figure 9: Exposure of the VIA by the Octopus System (43).

In terms of hospital morbidity and mortality, BC appears to be an encouraging approach compared with CEC (44).

An analysis of the STS ACSD from 2008 to 2011, on 25667 patients with an EF low (<30%) showed that the risks of death, stroke, and of major adverse cardiac events (MACCE) were lower in the beating heart group (45).

Analysis of the Japanese Adult Cardiovascular Surgery Database showed that CABG was associated with a reduction in early morbidity and mortality in patients with EF < 30% (46).

2- Duration of surgery :

Ait Houssa M et al (44), carried out a retrospective study comparing 2 groups of comparable patients with pre-operative left ventricular dysfunction: a group operated on with CEC, and a group operated on with CB. The duration of the operation was shorter in the beating heart group (p < 0.0001), but this was due to incomplete myocardial revascularisation in this group.

3- Revascularisation index :

According to t h e 2018 myocardial revascularisation recommendations (5), in the case of ostio-proximal IVA involvement, CABG is recommended in class IA. CB bypass could be a good alternative for the treatment of this type of lesion.However, in some studies, the rate of incomplete revascularisation is higher with the CB technique in patients with impaired LVEF, and this is due to the appearance of significant hypotension and poorly tolerated rhythm disturbances when the heart is dislocated, especially for anastomosis at the marginal (47).

Studies have shown that incomplete revascularisation increases the risk of MACCE and long-term mortality (15).

However, in a recent study by Kang et al, complete revascularisation had no benefit in terms of post-operative morbidity and mortality in multi-truncular patients with left ventricular dysfunction who had had a recent ST+ ACS (48).

4- Limits :

Coronary anastomoses are technically very difficult, as the surgeon is faced with problems of exposure and stabilisation of the anastomotic site (49).

In addition, myocardial revascularisation with CB is often incomplete in the bypass group, which could be the cause of a higher late mortality rate than in patients operated on with CEC (50). Also, complete surgical myocardial revascularisation improves late left ventricular function to a statistically significant extent in the CEC group (44). This haemodynamic improvement has an objective impact on quality of life. In the series by Ait Houssa et al (44), the authors observed more residual angina and more symptomatic patients in the BC group at follow-up. These opinions are shared by other authors (51).

IX-INTRAOPERATIVE CONVERSION TO BYPASS SURGERY

The STS (The Society of Thoracic Surgeons) database showed a conversion rate to bypass surgery of 5.2% for patients with impaired VF.Other studies have reported higher rates in association with impaired LVEF. And if the conversion was carried out as an emergency, the mortality rate was seven times higher. Another study reported that the hospital mortality rate increased from 5.4% to 32.1% in cases of conversion to emergency bypass (52, 53). Some teams prefer the beating heart technique in bypass surgery as a hybrid procedure, in order to achieve greater safety when performing anastomoses, and above all to achieve complete revascularisation and avoid emergency conversion. Recent studies have shown that this technique has been associated with a lower risk of postoperative morbidity and mortality in the short term compared with conventional bypass surgery under CEC (54, 55).

X- HYBRID CORONARY REVASCULARISATION

This is combined surgical and percutaneous coronary revascularisation. It consists of surgical revascularisation of the IVA by bypass using the AMIG, followed by percutaneous revascularisation of the other stenotic coronary arteries. This technique has not been widely adopted by the cardiovascular community, given the need for a hybrid operating theatre that allows operators to perform IVA bypass via a left mini-thoracotomy followed by angioplasty on the same day. However, this hybrid operating theatre is not available in most hospitals.A new approach was followed to facilitate the widespread use of the hybrid technique in multi-truncular patients with reduced left ventricular function, which consisted of performing the AMIG bypass on the IVA via median sternotomy and delaying percutaneous revascularisation to another time.

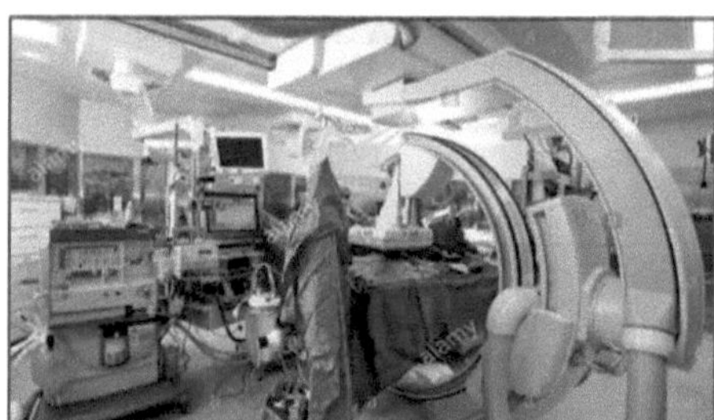

Figure 10: Hybrid operating room (56).

Minimally invasive techniques for bypassing the MIGA on the VIA have become increasingly attractive, fuelled by both the patient's and the doctors' desire to avoid the morbidity associated with median sternotomy and extracorporeal circulation. Currently, there are two commonly used robotic approaches that have proven their safety and efficacy: RA-MIDCAB (robotic-assisted minimally invasive coronary artery bypass) and TECAB (totally endoscopic coronary artery bypass). RA-MIDCAB offers the advantage of a direct hand-sewn anastomosis, but requires a 3 to 4 inch anterior thoracotomy and the ability to perform a beating heart anastomosis. This technique avoids the need for a thoracotomy, but requires the technical skill to perform a distal anastomosis by robot.Both techniques have been shown separately to be safe and effective in previous reports (57, 58). The study by Pasrija et al compared the two techniques and demonstrated similar survival and a similar incidence of post-operative complications. However, TECAB is a more expensive alternative, so a more thorough evaluation of post-operative pain, early rehabilitation and patient satisfaction is needed to determine whether an increase in costs is justified (59).

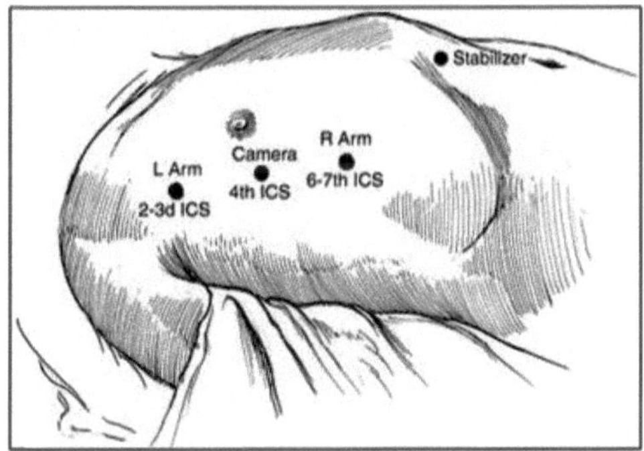

Figure 11: Trocar insertion sites; the location of the sites on the right for bypass of the CD and sometimes the IVA; the location of the sites on the left in mirror image for bypass of the IVA, Dg, Bx and Mg 1 or 2 (60).

XI-REVASCULARISATION UNDER CEC VERSUS REVASCULARISATION WITH CB

CEC is considered the gold standard in coronary revascularisation surgery. Several strategies have recently been used to reduce the complications associated with its use and to improve results (61). Techniques that do not use CEC have been shown to be safe and effective, even superior to conventional techniques in patients with ventricular dysfunction (62, 63). In the literature, patients operated on under CEC develop more post-operative complications and mortality. The study by Caputti et al (64) demonstrated a higher mortality rate, longer duration of mechanical ventilation, longer duration of hospitalisation in the intensive care unit and longer total hospitalisation in patients operated on by bypass graft. The incidence of post-operative complications such as bleeding, transfusion, bleeding recurrence, renal failure, haemodialysis and MI was lower in patients operated on with CB. These data were also demonstrated in the study by Buffolo et al (65).However, incomplete revascularisation is more common in BC surgery, which could reduce graft patency and long-term results.A large series of retrospective studies comparing patients with ventricular dysfunction who underwent revascularisation under CEC or CB failed to show differences between the two groups, suggesting that the CB procedure is safe and may lead to fewer complications despite the lack of statistically significant results. Furthermore, the results of surgery are highly dependent on the experience of the surgical team in the beating heart technique (66). Another recent study, the "CORONARY Trial" (67), which compared two groups of patients who underwent either CEC or CB surgery, showed that there was no significant difference in terms of results between the two groups. However, a meta-analysis (68) showed a higher mortality in patients operated on with CB, which could be due to a higher probability of graft occlusion or a higher rate of incomplete revascularisation.

XII- POST-OPERATIVE RESULTS

1- Operative mortality :

Left ventricular dysfunction is a major risk factor for perioperative morbidity and mortality in cardiac surgery patients. (69). In the literature, the operative mortality rate after myocardial revascularisation in patients with LV dysfunction is between 2.6% and 8.4% (12, 11). Hillis et al (13), in their study of 379 patients, concluded after a multivariate analysis that the factors predicting mortality were: age and chronic renal failure.In another study carried out by Nagendran et al (16) on 1326 patients, the factors predictive of mortality were: age, chronic renal failure, pre-operative LVEF < 35%, diabetes, peripheral arterial disease, redux surgery for CABG, recent MI, and TCG stenosis. The study by Isbir et al (70) of 1759 patients showed that chronic renal failure, age, LVEF ≤ 30%, PAH, recent MI, hypertension and the duration of aortic clamping were predictive factors of post-operative mortality.

Table III: Factors predictive of mortality according to the literature.

The study	Year	Number of patients	Factors predictive of mortality
Hillis et al (13)	1995-1999	379	Creator Cl< 45 ml/min/1.73 m2 Age
Nagendran et al (16)	1995-2008	1326	Age, CKD, LVEF <35%, diabetes, peripheral arterial disease, Redux, recent MI, TCG stenosis.
Isbir et al (70)	1996-2001	1759	Age, CKD, hypertension, LVEF ≤ 30%, PAPS> 40 mm Hg, high aortic clamping time.

2- Post-operative complications :

Myocardial infarction complicating coronary surgery is type 5 according to the universal definition (71).A review of the literature shows a postoperative MI rate of 2.7% after myocardial revascularisation under CEC in patients with preoperative ventricular dysfunction, and a rate of 0.95% in patients operated on with a beating heart (64). Stroke also remains a devastating complication after coronary artery bypass grafting (72). In the literature, the rate of stroke following coronary surgery has been reported to be 2.4% on average (73).

The incidence of mediastinitis varies according to the studies from 1 to 3% (extremes 0.5- 10%) after cardiac surgery by vertical median sternotomy (74). It complicates coronary surgery more than valvular or combined surgery (74).

Renal failure, which is included in the Euroscore II parameters and has been shown by various teams to be predictive of mortality, is a major complication in patients undergoing cardiac surgery. The rate of occurrence of infectious pneumonitis after myocardial revascularisation varies between 1.2% and 6.3% (75).Bleeding and blood transfusions are frequent surgical complications in patients undergoing coronary artery bypass grafting (76). Abundant bleeding or sudden onset of bleeding is a definite indication for repeat surgery, whether or not there are haemodynamic repercussions.

3- Use of tonic-cardiac drugs and Levosimendan :

Levosimendan is a compound used to treat heart failure and cardiogenic shock, and reduces the incidence of low cardiac output syndrome in patients with reduced LVEF after coronary artery bypass surgery (77). It has a positive inotropic effect without increasing myocyte energy requirements and vascular vasodilatory properties (78, 79). In the "LEVO-CTS" clinical trial, which is a multi-centre, randomised clinical trial including 882 patients with LVEF $\leq$ 35% undergoing coronary bypass, isolated mitral or aortic surgery, or combined surgery under CEC, the authors compared the effect of levosimendan with that of a placebo. There was no significant difference between the 2 groups in terms of early morbidity and mortality, but the 90-day mortality rate was significantly lower in the levosimendan group (80).

In a more recent study, of 848 patients with LV systolic dysfunction who underwent cardiac surgery, 563 patients underwent isolated coronary artery bypass grafting (283 patients received levosimendan and 280 patients received placebo) (81). The rate of mechanical circulatory assistance at 5 days and the mortality rate at 30 and 90 days were lower in the levosimendan group than in the placebo group (81).

The levosimendan group was associated with a statistically non-significant reduction in low cardiac output and inotrope use during the first 24 hours, and with a statistically significant reduction in mortality at 30 and 90 days compared with the placebo group.Eriksson et al (82) also demonstrated in their study that levosimendan improved cardiac output and facilitated weaning from bypass compared with placebo in 60 patients undergoing coronary bypass surgery. Tritapepe et al (83) also found that the use of levosimendan was accompanied by a significant reduction in troponin levels after coronary bypass surgery. In another study by Levin et al (84), patients who received levosimendan required lower doses of inotropes and vasopressors compared with patients who received placebo.

4- Post-operative mechanical circulatory support :

Its purpose is to provide uni or biventricular unloading, or to take over the entire workload of a failing heart that is not responding to optimal medical treatment. The current systems used to await recovery or heart transplantation are: the intra-aortic counterpulsation balloon (IACB), peristaltic roller pumps, external or internal assistance systems and ECMO (Extra-Corporeal Membrane Oxygenation). CPBIA is the most widely used because it can be introduced subcutaneously and is relatively inexpensive. The roller pump can only be used for a few hours, so its duration and effectiveness are limited, but it is useful in emergencies. As far as external assistance systems are concerned, external pneumatic ventricles connected to the Thoratec console are the most widely used in post-operative assistance for the treatment of certain cardiogenic shocks or while waiting for a heart transplant (85).

ECMO is a form of bypass surgery lasting several days, which can be used to treat acute circulatory and respiratory failure. The choice must take into account the patient, their pathology, the expected duration of assistance, the degree of urgency, the possibility of recovery of the assisted ventricle, uni- or biventricular failure, and the risk of haemorrhage and thromboembolism (60).

The current reasonable use of BCPIA is pre-operative support for patients in cardiogenic shock in preparation for revascularisation surgery after stabilisation and for improved post-operative recovery (86). Table IV shows the operative mortality rate and changes in LVEF. after revascularisation surgery in published series.

Table IV: The mean pre- and post-operative LVEF of patients with pre-operative left ventricular dysfunction and surgical revascularisation.

Study	Number of patients	Pre-operative LVEF (mean) (limits)	Operative mortality (%)	LVEF post-operative (average)	Improvement in post-operative LVEF (% of patients)
Elefteriades et al (11)	83	24,6% 10 à 30%	8,9%	33,2%	36%
Kron et al (12)	39	18,3% 10 à 20%	2,6%	26%	42%
Hillis et al (13)	379	28% 23 à 33%	5,5%	31%	-

The improvement in postoperative LVEF was statistically significant in the series by Elefteriades et al (11) (mean LVEF from 24.6% preoperatively to 33.2% postoperatively with p < 0.001), and in the series by Kron et al (mean LVEF from 18.7% preoperatively to 26% postoperatively with p < 0.05) (12, 13).

5- Late results :

In the series by Elefteriades et al (11), the survival rate was 87% at one year, 87% at 2 years and 80% at 3 years, and the majority of patients were NYHA stage I or II during their late follow-up. The 3-year survival rate was 80% in the series by Kron et al (12).

XIII- CONCLUSION

The number of coronary patients with impaired left ventricular (LV) systolic function proposed for coronary bypass surgery has increased in recent years. This combination of coronary artery disease and left ventricular dysfunction is associated with high post-operative mortality.Coronary artery bypass grafting (CABG) is an interesting alternative that may provide better preservation of postoperative ventricular function in these fragile patients, due to the absence of the inflammatory effects of extracorporeal circulation. However, this technique often results in incomplete myocardial revascularisation and a higher late mortality rate than in patients operated on using CEC. We are currently witnessing considerable development in revascularisation surgery techniques, especially in the case of a failing heart. One of the current challenges is to reduce the post-operative morbidity and mortality rate, which is still higher than that of surgery on a heart with good systolic function.Finally, a multi-disciplinary approach must be at the centre of the decision-making process for the treatment of coronary lesions with ventricular dysfunction, with the aim of developing a targeted revascularisation strategy. on the patient, and which should be at the heart of a discussion between cardiologists,interventional cardiologists, cardiac surgeons and anaesthetists.This 'heart team' approach should be based on risk scores for best therapeutic decision. However, surgery remains the gold standard for revascularisation in tritruncular patients or patients with TCG involvement in addition to ventricular dysfunction. The patient's opinion also remains essential and must be taken into account to guarantee truly informed and fair consent. Finally, other studies, mainly prospective, will enable us to study CABG on ventricular dysfunction more closely, to refine the indications and to guide the therapeutic decision in line with current recommendations.

BIBLIOGRAPHY

1- Ponikowski P, Voors AA, Anker SD, Bueno H, Cleland JGF, Coats AJS, et al. 2016 ESC Guidelines for the diagnosis and treatment of acute and chronic heart failure: The Task Force for the diagnosis and treatment of acute and chronic heart failure of the European Society of Cardiology (ESC)Developed with the special contribution of the Heart Failure Association (HFA) of the ESC. Eur Heart J. 14 July 2016; 37(27): 2129-200.

2- Vasan RS, Xanthakis V, Lyass A, Andersson C, Tsao C, Cheng S, et al. Epidemiology of Left Ventricular Systolic Dysfunction and Heart Failure in the Framingham Study. JACC: Cardiovascular Imaging. jan 2018;11(1):1‚11.

3- Gaziano TA. Cardiovascular Disease in the Developing World and Its Cost-Effective Management. Circulation. 6 Dec 2005;112(23):3547‚53.

4- Desai AS, Stevenson LW. Rehospitalization for Heart Failure: Predict or Prevent? Circulation. 24 Jul2012;126(4):501‚6.

5- Neumann F-J, Sousa-Uva M, Ahlsson A, Alfonso F, Banning AP, Benedetto U, et al. 2018 ESC/EACTS Guidelines on myocardial revascularization. European Heart Journal. 7 Jan 2019; 40(2):87‚165.

6- Shah S, Benedetto U, Caputo M, Angelini GD, Vohra HA. Comparison of the survival between coronary artery bypass graft surgery versus percutaneous coronary intervention in patients with poor left ventricular function (ejection fraction <30%): a propensity-matched analysis. European Journal of Cardio-Thoracic Surgery. 1 Feb 2019; 55(2): 238‚46.

7- Hassanabad AF, Mac Queen KT, Ali I. Surgical Treatment for Ischemic Heart Failure (STICH) trial: A review of outcomes. J Card Surg. Oct 2019; 34(10): 1075‚82.

8- Velazquez EJ, Lee KL, Jones RH, Al-Khalidi HR, Hill JA, Panza JA, et al.

Coronary-Artery Bypass Surgery in Patients with Ischemic Cardiomyopathy. N Engl J Med. 21 Apr 2016; 374(16): 1511̲20.

9- Sleilaty G, Achouh P, Fabiani J-N. Tritruncal coronary disease: angioplasty/stent or coronary artery bypass grafts? Current status and review of the literature. Annales de Cardiologie et d'Angéiologie. Apr 2009; 58(2): 104̲12.

10- Tiquet B, Blossier JD, Orsel I, Pihan F, Piccardo A, Marsaud JP, et al. Short-Term Outcomes After Off-Pump or On-Pump Coronary Artery Bypass Grafting in the Octogenarian Patients. J Cardiothorac Vasc Anesth. Jul 2019; 33(7): 2100̲2.

11- Elefteriades JA, Tolis G, Levi E, et al. Coronary artery bypass grafting in severe left ventricular dysfunction: excellent survival with improved ejection fraction and functional state. J Am Coll Cardiol 1993; 22: 1411-1417.

12- Kron IL, Flanagan TL, Blackbourne LH, Schroeder RA, Nolan SP. Coronary Revascularization Rather than Cardiac Transplantation for Chronic Ischemic Cardiomyopathy: Annals of Surgery. Sept 1989; 210(3): 348̲54.

13- Hillis GS. Outcome of Patients With Low Ejection Fraction Undergoing Coronary Artery Bypass Grafting: Renal Function and Mortality After 3.8 Years. Circulation. 4 Jul 2006; 114(1_suppl): I-414-I-419.

14- Wu F-Y, Lu Y-C, Lai S-T, Weng Z-C, Huang C-H. Coronary Artery Bypass Grafting in Patients with Left Ventricular Dysfunction. Journal of the Chinese Medical Association. May 2006; 69(5): 218-23.

15- Wang W, Wang Y, Piao H, Li B, Wang T, Li D, et al. Early and Medium Outcomes of On-Pump Beating-Heart versus Off-Pump CABG in Patients with Moderate Left Ventricular Dysfunction. Braz J Cardiovasc Surg [Internet]. 2019 [cited 28 Jan 2020]; 34 (1). Available from: https://bjcvs.org/pdf/3059/v34n1a12.pdf.

16- Nagendran J, Norris CM, Graham MM, Ross DB, Mac Arthur RG, Kieser

TM, et al. Coronary Revascularization for Patients With Severe Left Ventricular Dysfunction. The Annals of Thoracic Surgery. Dec 2013; 96(6): 2038-44.

17- Nagendran J, Bozso SJ, Norris CM, Mc Alister FA, Appoo JJ, Moon MC, et al. Coronary Artery Bypass Surgery Improves Outcomes in Patients With Diabetes and Left Ventricular Dysfunction. Journal of the American College of Cardiology. Feb 2018; 71(8): 819-27.

18- Barstow C, Rice M, Mc Divitt JD. Acute coronary syndrome: diagnostic evaluation. Am Fam Physician. 1 Feb 2017;95(3):170-7.

19- Algarni KD, Elhenawy AM, Maganti M, Collins S, Yau TM. Decreasing prevalence but increasing importance of left ventricular dysfunction and reoperative surgery in prediction of mortality in coronary artery bypass surgery: Trends over 18 years. The Journal of Thoracic and Cardiovascular Surgery. August 2012; 144(2): 340-346.e1.

20 Sousa-Uva M, Alfonso F, Banning AP, Benedetto U, Byrne RA, Collet J-P, et al. The Task Force on myocardial revascularization of the European Society of Cardiology (ESC) and European Association for Cardio-Thoracic Surgery (EACTS): 96.

21- Blazek S, Rossbach C, Borger MA, Fuernau G, Desch S, Eitel I, et al. Comparison of Sirolimus-Eluting Stenting With Minimally Invasive Bypass Surgery for Stenosis of the Left Anterior Descending Coronary Artery. JACC Cardiovasc Interv. Jan 2015; 8(1): 308.

22- Houlind K, Kjeldsen BJ, Madsen SN, Rasmussen BS, Holme SJ, Nielsen PH, et al. On-Pump Versus Off-Pump Coronary Artery Bypass Surgery in Elderly patients: Results From the Danish On-Pump Versus Off-Pump Randomization Study. Circulation. May 22, 2012; 125(20): 24319.

23- Raja SG, Dreyfus GD. Impact of off-pump coronary artery bypass surgery on postoperative pulmonary dysfunction: current best available evidence. Ann

Card Anaesth. Jan 2006; 9(1): 17-24.

24- Lev-Ran O, Loberman D, Matsa M, Pevni D, Nesher N, Mohr R, et al. Reduced strokes in the elderly: the benefits of untouched aorta off-pump coronary surgery. Ann Thorac Surg. Jan 2004; 77(1): 102-7.

25- Edelman JJ, Yan TD, Padang R, Bannon PG, Vallely MP. Off-pump coronary artery bypass surgery versus percutaneous coronary intervention: a meta-analysis of randomized and nonrandomized studies. Ann Thorac Surg. Oct 2010; 90(4): 1384-90.

26- Beauford RB, Saunders CR, Lunceford TA, Niemeier LA, Shah S, Karanam R, et al. Multivessel off-pump revascularization in patients with significant left main coronary artery stenosis: early and midterm outcome analysis. J Card Surg. Apr 2005; 20(2): 112-8.

27- Kerr PC, Ricci M, Abraham R, D'Ancona G, Salerno TA. Redo left anterior descending artery grafting via left anterior small thoracotomy: an alternative approach. Ann Thorac Surg. Jan 2001; 71(1): 384-5.

28- Bonchek LI, lJllyot DJ. Minimally invasive coronary bypass. A dissenting opinion [editorial]. Circulation 1998; 98: 495-7.

29- Ling Y, Bao L, Yang W, Chen Y, Gao Q. Minimally invasive direct coronary artery bypass grafting with an improved rib spreader and a new-shaped cardiac stabilizer: results of 200 consecutive cases in a single institution. BMC Cardiovasc Disord. Dec 2016; 16(1): 42.

30- Blanc P, Aouifi A, Chiari P, Bouvier H, Jegaden O, Lehot J.J. Minimally invasive cardiac surgery: surgical techniques and anaesthetic features. Ann Fr Anesth Réanim1999; 18: 748-71.

31- Gulielmos V, Knaut M, Wagner FM, Schtiler S. Minimally invasive surgical technique for the treatment of multivessel coronary artery disease. Ann Thorac Surg 1998; 65: 1331-4.

32- Ramachandra C. Reddy. Minimally invasive direct coronary artery bypass:

Technical considerations. Semin Thoracic Surg 2011; 23: 216-219.

33- Hartz RS. On behalf of the Executive Committee of the Council on Cardio-Thoracic and Vascular Surgery. Minimally invasive heart surgery. Circulation 1996; 94: 2669-70.

34- Magruder JT, Young A, Grimm JC, Conte JV, Shah AS, Mandal K, et al. Bilateral internal thoracic artery grafting: Does graft configuration affect outcome? J Thorac Cardiovasc Surg. Jul 2016; 152(1): 120-7.

35- Acuff TE, Landreneau RJ, Griffith BP, Mack MJ. Minimally invasive coronary artery bypass grafting. Ann Thorac Surg 1996; 61: 135-7.

36- Arslan U, Calik E, Tekin AI, Erkut B. Off-pump versus on-pump complete coronary artery bypass grafting: Comparison of the effects on the renal damage in patients with renal dysfunction. Medicine. August 2018; 97(35): e12146.

37- Florisson DS, De Bono JA, Davies RA, Newcomb AE. Doesminimally invasive coronary artery bypass improve outcomes compared to off-pump coronary bypass via sternotomy in patients undergoing coronary artery bypass grafting? Interact Cardiovasc Thorac Surg. 01 2018; 27(3): 357-64.

38- Akins CW. Mini-CABG: a step forward or a step backward? The " con " point of view. J Cardio thorac Vast Anesth 1997; 11: 669-72.

39- Vallely MP, Bannon PG, Bayfield MS, Hughes CF, Kritharides L. Quantitative and temporal differences in coagulation, fibrinolysis and platelet activation after on-pump and off-pump coronary artery bypass surgery. Heart Lung Circ Apr 2009; 18(2): 123,30.

40- Lev-Ran O, Loberman D, Matsa M, Pevni D, Nesher N, Mohr R, et al. Reduced strokes in the elderly: the benefits of untouched aorta off-pump coronary surgery. Ann Thorac Surg. Jan 2004; 77(1): 102,7.

41- AromKV, Emery; RW, Nicoloff DM, Flavin TF, Emery AM. Minimally invasive direct coronary artery bypass grafting: experimental and clinical experiences. Ann Thorac Surg 1997; 63: 48-52.

42- Gu YJ, Mariani MA. Van Oeveren W, Grandjean JG. Boonstra PW. Reduction of the inflammatory response in patients undergoing minimally invasive coronary artery bypass grafting. Ann Thorac Surg 1998; 65: 420-4.

43- PAC - Précis of cardiac anaesthesia [Internet]. [cited 20 Feb 2020].

Available at:

http://www.precisdanesthesiecardiaque.ch/Chapitre10/Pontagaortocoron.html.

44- Ait Houssa M, Moutakiallah Y, Abdou A, Selkane C, Amahzoune B, Drissi M, et al. Results of coronary bypass in left ventricular dysfunction (comparison of beating heart and CEC). Annals of Cardiology and Aneiology. August 2013; 62(4): 2417.

45- Jarral OA, Saso S, Athanasiou T. Off-pump coronary artery bypass in patients with left ventricular dysfunction: a meta-analysis. Ann Thorac Surg. Nov 2011; 92(5): 168694.

46- Ueki C, Miyata H, Motomura N, Sakaguchi G, Akimoto T, Takamoto S. Off- pump versus on-pump coronary artery bypass grafting in patients with left ventricular dysfunction. J Thorac Cardiovasc Surg. Apr 2016; 151(4): 10928.

47- Khan H, Uzzaman M, Benedetto U, Butt S, Raja SG. On- or off-pump coronary artery bypass grafting for octogenarians: a meta-analysis of comparative studies involving 27,623 patients. Int J Surg. 2017; 47: 42-51.

48- Kang J, Zheng C, Park KW, Park J, Rhee T, Lee HS, et al. Complete Revascularization of Multi-vessel Coronary Artery Disease Does Not Improve Clinical Outcome in ST-Segment Elevation Myocardial Infarction Patients with Reduced Left Ventricular Ejection Fraction. JCM. 15 Jan 2020; 9(1): 232.

49- Gulielmos V, Knaut M, Wagner FM, Schtiler S. Minimally invasive surgical technique for the treatment of multivessel coronary artery disease. Ann Thorac

Surg 1998; 65: 1331-4.

50- Jarral OA, Saso S, Athanasiou T. Off-pump coronary artery bypass in patients with left ventricular dysfunction: a meta-analysis. Ann Thorac Surg. Nov 2011; 92(5): 1686 94.

51- Bull DA, Neumayer LA, Stringham JC, Meldrum P, Affleck DG, Karwande SV. Coronary bypass grafting with cardiopulmonary bypass versus off-pump cardiopulmonary bypass grafting: does eliminating the pump reduce morbidity and cost? Ann Thorac Surg 2001; 71: 170-5.

52- Mishra M, Shrivastava S, Dhar A, Bapna R, Mishra A, Meharwal ZS, et al. A prospective evaluation of hemodynamic instability during off-pump coronary artery bypass surgery. J Cardiothorac Vasc Anesth. 2003; 17(4): 452-8.

53- Maroto Castellanos LC, Carnero M, Cobiella FJ, Alswies A, Ayaon A, Reguillo FJ, et al. Off-pump to on-pump emergency conversion: incidence, risk factors, and impact on short- and long-term results. J Card Surg. 2015; 30(10): 735-45.

54- Miyahara K, Matsuura A, Takemura H, Saito S, Sawaki S, Yoshioka T, et al. On-pump beating-heart coronary artery bypass grafting after acute myocardial infarction has lower mortality and morbidity. J Thorac Cardiovasc Surg. 2008; 135(3): 521-6.

55- Passaroni AC, Felicio ML, Campos NLKL, Silva MAM, Yoshida WB. Hemolysis and inflammatory response to extracorporeal circulation during on-pump CABG: comparison between roller and centrifugal pump systems. Braz J Cardiovasc Surg. 2018; 33(1): 64-71.

56- Limited, A. Cardiac surgery in a hybrid operating theatre, Deutsches Herzzentrum Berlin or German Heart Centre, Berlin, Germany, Europe Ban Images, Photo Stock: 279532311.Alamy https://www.alamyimages.fr/chirurgie-cardiaque-dans-une-salle-d-operation- hybrid-deutsches-herzzentrum-berlin-or-cardiac-centre-german-berlin- germany-europe-image 279532311.html.

57- Yang M, Wu Y, Wang G, Xiao C, Zhang H, Gao C. Robotic total arterial off-pump coronary artery bypass grafting: seven-year single-center experience and long-term follow-up of graft patency. Ann Thorac Surg. 2015; 100: 1367-1373.

58- Halkos ME, Liberman HA, Devireddy C, et al. Early clinical and angiographic outcomes after robotic-assisted coronary artery bypass surgery. J Thorac Cardiovasc Surg. 2014; 147: 179-185.

59- Pasrija C, Kon ZN, Ghoreishi M, Lehr EJ, Gammie JS, Griffith BP, et al. Cost and Outcome of Minimally Invasive Techniques for Coronary Surgery Using Robotic Technology. Innovations (Phila). Jul 2018; 13(4): 282-6.

60- Cannesson M, Bastien O, Lehot J. Particularities of haemodynamic management after cardiac surgery. Réanimation. Mai 2005; 14(3): 216-24.

61- Darwazah AK, Bader V, Isleem I, Helwa K. Myocardial revascularization using on-pump beating heart among patients with left ventricular dysfunction. J Cardiothorac Surg. 2010; 5: 109.

62- Youn YN, Chang BC, Hong YS, Kwak YL, Yoo KJ. Early and mid-term impacts of cardiopulmonary bypass on coronary artery bypass grafting in patients with poor left ventricular dysfunction: a propensity score analysis. Circ J. 2007; 71: 1387-94.

63- Darwazah AK, Abu Sham'a RA, Hussein E, Hawari MH, Ismail H. Myocardial revascularization in patients with low ejection fraction: effect of pump technique on early morbidity and mortality. J Card Surg 2006; 21: 22-7.

64- Caputti GM, Palma JH, Gaia DF, Buffolo E. Off-pump coronary artery bypass surgery in selected patients is superior to the conventional approach for patients with severely depressed left ventricular function. Clinics (Sao Paulo). Dec 2011; 66(12): 2049-53.

65- Buffolo E, Branco JN, Gerola LR, Aguiar LF, Teles CA, Palma JH, et al. Off- pump myocardial revascularization: critical analysis of 23 years' experience in 3,866 patients. Ann Thorac Surg. 2006; 81: 85-9.

66- Shroyer AL, Grover FL, Hattler B, Collins JF, McDonald GO, Kozora E, et al. On-pump versus off-pump coronary-artery bypass surgery. N Engl J Med. 2009; 361: 1827-37.

67- Lamy A, Devereaux PJ, Prabhakaran D, Taggart DP, Hu S, Straka Z, et al. Five-Year Outcomes after Off-Pump or On-Pump Coronary-Artery Bypass Grafting. N Engl J Med. 15 Dec 2016; 375(24): 2359‑68.

68- Takagi H, Matsui M, Umemoto T. Off-pump coronary artery bypass may increase late mortality: a meta-analysis of randomized trials. Ann Thorac Surg. 2010; 89: 1881-8.

69- Topkara VK, Cheema FH, Kesavaramanujam S, Mercando ML, Cheema AF, Namerow PB, et al. Coronary artery bypass grafting in patients with low ejection fraction. Circulation. 2005; 112: I344-50.

70- Selim Isbir C, Yildirim T, Akgun S, Civelek A, Aksoy N, Oz M, et al. Coronary artery bypass surgery in patients with severe left ventricular dysfunction. International Journal of Cardiology. August 2003; 90(2‑3): 309‑16.

71- Thygesen K, Alpert JS, Jaffe AS, Chaitman BR, Bax JJ, Morrow DA, et al. Fourth universal definition of myocardial infarction (2018). European Heart Journal. 14 Jan 2019; 40(3): 237‑69.

72- Almassi GH, Sommers T, Moritz TE, Shroyer AL, London MJ, Henderson WG, et al. Stroke in cardiac surgical patients: determinants and outcome. Ann Thorac Surg. August 1999; 68(2): 391‑7; discussion 397-398.

73- Muneretto C, Negri A, Manfredi J, Terrini A, Rodella G, Elqarra S, et al. Safety and usefulness of composite grafts for total arterial myocardial revascularization: a prospective randomized evaluation. J Thorac Cardio vasc

Surg. Apr 2003; 125(4): 826-35.

74- Lemaignen A, Birgand G, Ghodhbane W, Alkhoder S, Lolom I, Belorgey S, et al. Sternal wound infection after cardiac surgery: incidence and risk factors according to clinical presentation. Clin Microbiol Infect Off Publ Eur Soc Clin Microbiol Infect Dis. Jul 2015;21(7): 674.e11-18.

75- Robinson BM, Paterson HS, Denniss AR. Composite Y-Grafting Using the Left Internal Thoracic Artery: Survival and Angiography in 198 Cases. Heart, Lung and Circulation. Jul 2017; 26(7): 7249.

76- Munoz JJ, Birkmeyer NJ, Birkmeyer JD, O'Connor GT, Dacey LJ. Is epsilon-amino caproic acid as effective as a protinin in reducing bleeding with cardiac surgery : ameta-analysis. Circulation. 5 Jan 1999; 99(1): 819.

77- Yoon Y-H, Ahn J-M, Kang D-Y, Park H, Cho S-C, Lee PH, et al. Impact of SYNTAX Score on 10-Year Outcomes After Revascularization for Left Main Coronary Artery Disease. JACC: Cardiovascular Interventions. Feb 2020; 13(3): 36171.

78- Toller W, Heringlake M, Guarracino F, Algotsson L, Alvarez J, Argyriadou H, et al. Preoperative and perioperative use of levosimendan in cardiac surgery: European expert opinion. Int J Cardiol 2015; 184: 323-36.

79- Michaels AD, McKeown B, Kostal M, Vakharia KT, Jordan MV, Gerber IL, et al. Effects of intravenous levosimendan on human coronary vasomotor regulation, left ventricular wall stress, and myocardial oxygen uptake. Circulation. 2005; 111: 1504-9.

80- Mehta RH, Van Diepen S, Meza J, Bokesch P, Leimberger JD, Tourt-Uhlig S, et al. Levosimendan in patients with left ventricular systolic dysfunction undergoing cardiac surgery on cardiopulmonary bypass: rationale and study design of the levosimendan in patients with left ventricular systolic dysfunction undergoing cardiac surgery requiring cardiopulmonary bypass (LEVO-CTS) trial. Am Heart J. 2016; 182: 62-71.

81- Van Diepen S, Mehta RH, Leimberger JD, Goodman SG, Fremes S, Jankowich R, Heringlake M, Anstrom KJ, Levy JH, Luber J, Nagpal AD, Duncan AE, Argenziano M, Toller W, Teoh K, Knight JD, Lopes RD, Cowper PA, Mark DB, and Alexander JH. Levosimendan in patients with reduced left ventricular function undergoing isolated coronary or valve surgery. The Journal of Thoracic and Cardiovascular Surgery 2019; 145: 56-63.

82- Eriksson HI, Jalonen JR, Heikkinen LO, Kivikko M, Laine M, Leino KA, et al. Levosimendan facilitates weaning from cardiopulmonary bypass in patients undergoing coronary artery bypass grafting with impaired left ventricular function. Ann Thorac Surg. 2009; 87: 448-54.

83- Tritapepe L, De Santis V, Vitale D, Guarracino F, Pellegrini F, Pietropaoli P, et al. Levosimendan pre-treatment improves outcomes in patients undergoing coronary artery bypass graft surgery. Br J Anaesth. 2009; 102: 198-204.

84- Levin R, Degrange M, Del Mazo C, Tanus E, Porcile R. Preoperative levosimendan decreases mortality and the development of low cardiac output in high-risk patients with severe left ventricular dysfunction undergoing coronary artery bypass grafting with cardiopulmonary bypass. Exp Clin Cardiol. 2012; 17: 125-30.

85- Mehta S, Aufiero T, Pae WJ, Miller C, Pierce X. Combined registry for the clinical use of mechanical ventricular assist pumps and the total artificial heart in conjunction with heart transplantation: sixth official report. J Heart Transplant 1995; 14: 585-93.

86- Maeda K, Takanashi S, Saiki Y. Perioperative use of the intra-aortic balloon pump: where do we stand in 2018? Current Opinion in Cardiology. Nov 2018; 33(6): 61321.

TABLE OF CONTENTS

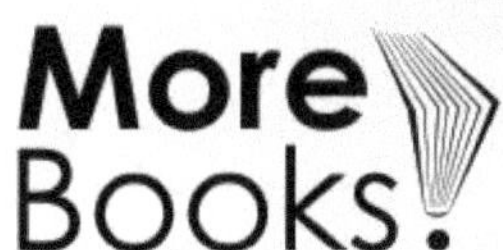

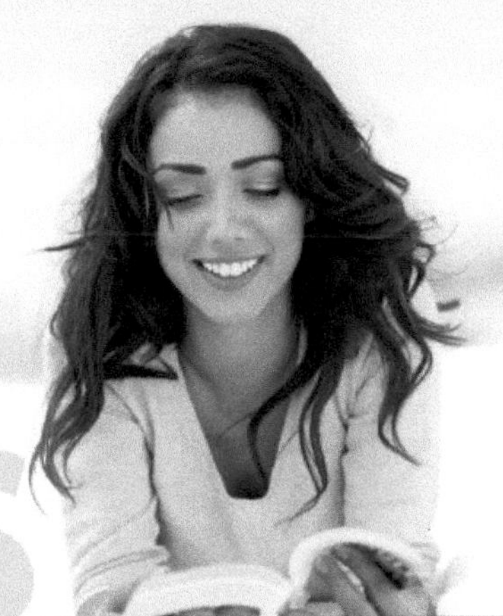

yes **I want** morebooks!

Buy your books fast and straightforward online - at one of world's fastest growing online book stores! Environmentally sound due to Print-on-Demand technologies.

Buy your books online at
www.morebooks.shop

Kaufen Sie Ihre Bücher schnell und unkompliziert online – auf einer der am schnellsten wachsenden Buchhandelsplattformen weltweit! Dank Print-On-Demand umwelt- und ressourcenschonend produzi ert.

Bücher schneller online kaufen
www.morebooks.shop

info@omniscriptum.com
www.omniscriptum.com

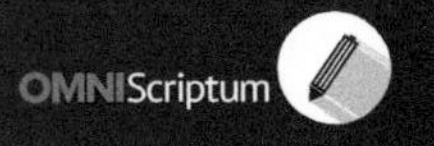

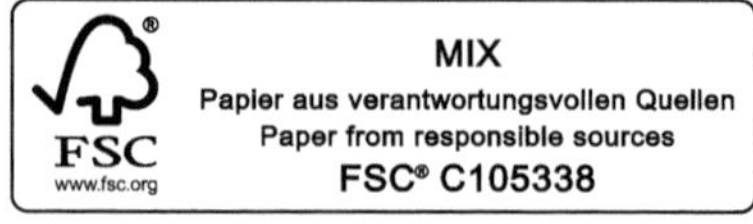

Printed by Books on Demand GmbH, Norderstedt / Germany